Q

S

V

W

Y

X

Z

B

A

C

d

E

h

F

g

A

IS FOR

ADVICE

the reassuring kind

MORROW
GIFT

An Imprint of WILLIAM MORROW

A

IS FOR

ADVICE

the reassuring kind

WISDOM FOR PREGNANCY

ILANA STANGER-ROSS

For all the families
I've had the honor to work
with — thank you

INTRODUCTION

The evening after I shyly shared news of my first pregnancy with my sister-in-law, I came home from work to find a bag of well-worn books on my doorstep. The bag held every bestselling pregnancy advice book, and I sat down eager to consume them all. But as I flipped through the pages, disappointment settled in. A few of the books outlined every potential pregnancy disorder and disaster; others advocated for a particular kind of birth. Eventually I stacked them all in a neat little pile where they sat for the rest of my pregnancy. I didn't want to be told all that could go wrong, or the only way to do things right. I just wanted old-fashioned reassurance—to be told that it would be okay, to be reminded that I wasn't alone.

At the same time as I became a mother, I enrolled in the midwifery program at the University of British Columbia in Vancouver, Canada. In most Canadian provinces, midwifery is fully integrated into the health-care system; in Victoria, British Columbia, where I now practice, midwives attend over 30 percent of deliveries, working alongside our nursing, family physician, obstetrician, and pediatrician colleagues.

Three children, one four-year Canadian midwifery degree, and hundreds of births later, I am writing the stories that I wanted to read—and that my clients, through their questions, ask me to tell them.

This book is for anyone who has experienced the transformation of pregnancy—in your own body or the body of someone you love. I've addressed it to first-time parents, but I hope it will speak to you wherever you are in your pregnancy journey—the first time or the fifth, overjoyed, ambivalent, terrified, or all of the above.

While I write from a place of reassurance, I don't mean to advocate complacency. Despite having the costliest maternity care system in the world, the U.S. maternal mortality rate is higher than that of any other developed nation. There are massive racial disparities in health outcomes: African American women are three to four times more likely to die in or after childbirth, even when controlling for income and socioeconomic status. By demanding that pregnancy and childbirth be a journey marked by informed and supportive care providers, this book also represents a call to action.

Every pregnant person deserves to be well cared for in pregnancy, during labor and delivery, and throughout the postpartum period. I hope the stories in this book bring comfort and instill strength for that most important story of all: your own.

A
IS FOR
ADVICE

the reassuring kind

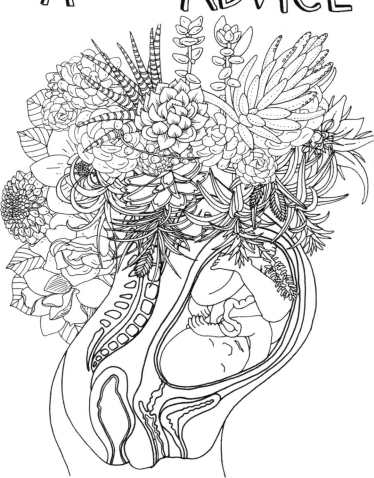

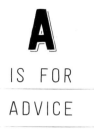

A

IS FOR

ADVICE

There was a time when birth was all around us. It took place nearby, in the home, in the village. There was no need to go hunting for advice manuals to explain what would happen—the knowledge was oral, witnessed, and passed down. Talismans offered protection, ceremonies promised order. The grandmother could help latch the baby, the aunt could demonstrate a swaddle.

This isn't about romanticizing the past or the developing world. Birth is never ordinary. Talismans were there for a reason; nature can be cruel.

We have gained so much. We are so lucky to birth in a time and place where we can access trained care providers, drugs, operating rooms, blood.

And yet: we have lost something too. Most of us will have never seen a birth before giving birth ourselves, and that vacuum fuels our fear. We search for meaningful reassurance at a time when, though childbirth has never been safer, every film and television show depicts birth as an emergency.

"Push!" the television doctor yells in a scene so well-worn that likely we can all script the rest on cue: the teary-eyed father trying to be brave; the desperate mother saying no, no, I can't do it; the concerned nurse reporting something about oxygen or blood or heart rate patterns; the doctor, even more urgent now, screaming "Push! Push!"—and then, just when all seems lost, the triumphant last red-faced effort, the baby's cry, the mother's tears.

And enter the perfectly swaddled six-month-old baby.

(Perhaps the lesson of these television and film depictions of birth really should be: it's always dangerous to try to birth a six-month-old.)

Even worse are the stories that so many women share with pregnant friends. When I was pregnant with my first child and introduced to this genre, I dubbed it "Tales of Miscarriage and Mayhem." It's not that I advocate silencing those who have had difficult experiences: those stories matter. But as a pregnant woman I heard more "she almost died" than "everything went really well," and I wondered why so many women seemed so set on, well, scaring me.

And then there's the consumerism of modern-day pregnancy: strollers and car seats; cribs, bassinets, and baby wraps; diaper and monitor systems; developmentally appropriate toys and safety locks and . . . and in this way, one of the most profound passages in a person's life can quickly be reduced to a surprisingly stressful shopping experience.

And yet: pregnancy, birth, those first exhausting weeks of parenting—what an amazing time-out-of-time. What happens when a woman becomes a mother happens both to her and through her. She is both the traveler and the road traveled and her journey, however it unfolds, will have meaning for her for a lifetime.

Pregnancy advice books generally come with the warning that they're not meant to replace the advice of a medical professional. To mine I will add: this book isn't meant to replace pregnancy advice books. I won't offer a month-by-month guide to gestation, or a detailed overview of pregnancy disorders. Instead, I'll give the advice that I share with my own midwifery clients—not the clinical recommendations or informed-choice discussions that I provide on a regular basis, but the advice that creeps into the corners of conversation, the words I say when they ask for more.

Some advice on advice, then: choose carefully what you listen to. And as you travel through the exhaustion and the hassle, the fear and the unpredictability, remember to laugh, and to reflect, and to spend some time just marveling at the wonder of it all.

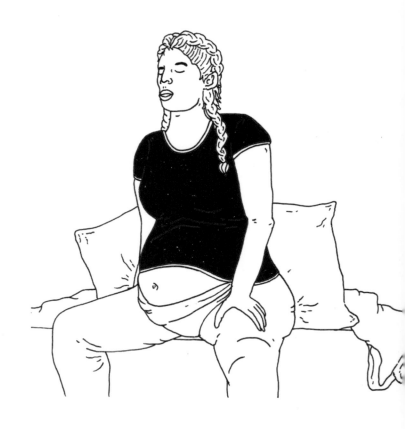

B is for Breath

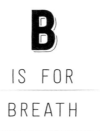

IS FOR

BREATH

I promise that I am not about to give you a detailed list of breathing instructions.

But, while there are very few universal truths in labor, here's one: almost every woman panics at some point.

And sometimes a gentle reminder to take a deep breath releases that tension.

As with labor so with everything in life: breathe. Deep, slow, and once again: breathe. It's a cliché, sure. But for good reason.

It's not that you can breathe your way to a perfect birth and a perfect baby.

I wish it were that easy, but it isn't.

But you can trick yourself past panic by taking full, deep breaths. Breaths that remind you where you are and what your job is at that moment, whether it's remaining at home in the early hours of labor despite an urge to rush to the hospital, or closing your eyes against the glare of the operating room lights as you open yourself to a surgical birth, or knees-bent pushing from a place so deep inside you never knew it existed before.

sometimes a gentle reminder to take a deep breath releases tension

Or now, as you read this book and wonder, perhaps with excitement or perhaps with trepidation, what your story will be.

Or later, when the baby is crying and your body is sore and you find yourself feeling, maybe, just a little bit lost.

Breathe.

It's not a solution. It's just the first step. Breathe to remind yourself that you matter, that you are worthy, that you are trying your best.

The journey from pregnancy to parenthood can be joyful, wonderful, terrible, exhausting, exhilarating, and all of the above.

It is a profound journey.

Learn this lesson now and it will serve you again and again.

Breathe. Deep and full, in and out, slow and steady.

Try it.

No, really. C'mon: try it. Breathe: deep and full, in and out, slow and steady.

No one will notice.

Breathe in strength, and breathe out forgiveness.

And then keep it up as needed for, well, forever.

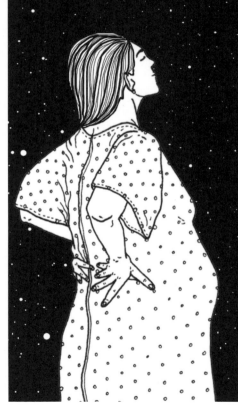

C IS FOR CONTROL

C

IS FOR

CONTROL

I once overheard one of my midwifery colleagues speaking to an expectant couple. "Birth is about surrendering to the unknown," she told them.

I liked that phrase, and promptly stole it from her.

Many women—maybe most women—fear this surrender. They see it as a loss of control.

They ask, Should I write a birth plan? Will that help?

Maybe. Educating yourself about your options, about what or what might not be routine for your care provider or your place of birth, makes sense.

So, too, does reflecting on what matters most to you and sharing these thoughts with whoever will be supporting you during labor.

But here is the thing: you cannot control your birth.

Here is the other thing: you will always be you. You won't lose yourself, though you might find yourself making some noises that are new to you.

Letting go can be okay. When a friend makes you laugh so much you snort—that's a loss of control. When we open ourselves to grief and sob out our anguish—that's a loss of control too.

Some of life's most meaningful moments depend on our surrender.

But here's the very important thing that I ask every woman to remember, and it's so important that I am going to stick it on its own line and start it off with a capital letter:

Loss of control does not mean loss of consent.

You cannot control your birth. There are too many unknowns. You can know everything and prepare for everything, and still you may find that your body and your baby don't cooperate as you wish they would have.

But nothing should happen to you or your baby without your informed consent.

This applies to: everything. To each internal exam, to any IV or injection, and to any suggestion of an assisted (with forceps or a vacuum) or operative (cesarean section) birth. Hospitals have consent forms for surgeries, but real consent means more than signing a form—it means understanding why a care provider thinks that intervention is the best course, and agreeing to that recommendation.

The first birth I ever attended ended in a cesarean section. I was a first-year midwifery student, eight months pregnant and wonderfully optimistic. The laboring woman, Jaqueline, was a first-time mom as well. The midwife and I assessed her after a long early labor: her baby was still high, her cervix still thick, and when her water had broken, just prior to our arrival, it was brown flecked rather than clear—her baby had been a bit too precocious and pooped while still in utero, which can be a sign of stress. Though she'd been hoping for a home birth, she readily agreed to a hospital transfer; once there, at the midwife's recommendation, she received an epidural for rest and pain relief and Pitocin to promote stronger, more coordinated contractions.

I don't remember when the midwife first mentioned the possibility of a cesarean section, but I do remember thinking: Why is she bringing that up now? It seemed to me that we should be encouraging Jaqueline, and that mentioning a C-section was resigning her to that outcome. What was the role of hope? I wondered. Why was the midwife so pessimistic?

Afterward—after the surgery, and my first postbirth nap—I did some research. I was curious about what makes a "good" birth experience. What I found surprised me and helped me understand why the midwife had mentioned a cesarean section when she did.

Those who report the most positive birth experiences aren't necessarily the ones who have what you might consider a textbook "normal" birth.

Instead, the women who report the most positive birth experiences are those who feel they understood all decisions made and had a say in the decision-making process. That holds even for complicated births among women who had been hoping for "natural" deliveries—births that require multiple interventions, births that end in surgery.

In many births—in much of medicine—there's a balance to be achieved between encouraging and informing. Finding that balance is art rather than science, and every care provider struggles, sometimes, to get it right.

Jaqueline did well postpartum. She was disappointed that her birth hadn't gone as she hoped, but reflecting on it she said, "I understand."

I thought of Jaqueline a few years ago when Brenda, a second-time mom, came to me hoping for a vaginal birth after a previous cesarean (VBAC). She'd found her first cesarean section difficult and cried as she told me about it. Due to pregnancy complications, her labor had been induced at thirty-seven weeks gestation. But her baby hadn't tolerated the induction, and Brenda had quickly been transferred to the OR.

For Brenda, the hardest part had been the surprise of it. Suddenly she was being rushed across the hall, and she hadn't prepared for that possibility.

Many months later, when Brenda was close to delivery and recounting her story again, I asked whether anyone had warned her that as a first-time mom being induced at thirty-seven weeks she had a significantly increased risk of cesarean section.

"No," she told me. "No one said anything."

And yet: her care provider would have known. Perhaps

the care provider had wanted to encourage Brenda; perhaps she hadn't wanted to disappoint her. And perhaps she had mentioned the increased surgical risk, but Brenda just wasn't able to hear her.

Would Brenda's experience have been different if she had understood the facts?

I think it would have. Though she wouldn't have had any more control over the outcome, she would have been able to provide truly informed consent.

People will say: but emergencies happen, you can't always have a long discussion of risks and benefits.

It is true that things can change quickly in birth. But those moments of fast-paced action are far less common than people might think. Most of the time there is time to ensure that a woman has provided informed consent.

As for the true emergencies—when urgent care is needed, a room can fill up quickly. The woman may never have met the nurses and specialists who must quickly assume care of her and her baby. But if she has been treated with respect by her primary care provider, if she has trusted that person's actions, then hopefully she will trust the decision made by that caregiver—midwife or doctor or nurse—to call in the full team, to act swiftly together.

You cannot control your birth. (Or your child, for that matter.) But you can ensure that your voice stays at the center of your birth story. Consent matters.

Make sure it matters to your care provider, too.

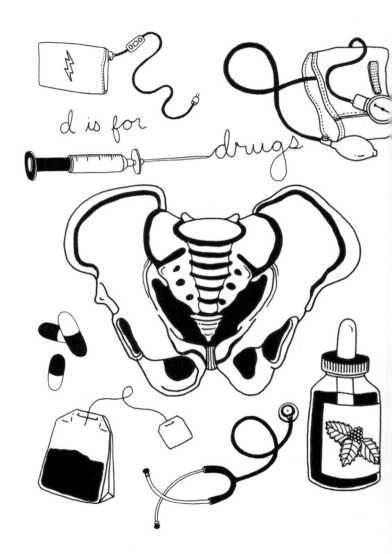

d is for drugs

D

IS FOR

DRUGS

"I want an epidural," Tracey tells me. Her voice is firm, just shy of challenging. She chose midwifery care for the longer visits and the extra postpartum support, but she wants me to know—experiencing pain is not part of her plan.

"There is no way I am having an epidural," Jessica says. She is planning a home birth, and she is emphatic: she wants no interventions.

Pop-quiz time. An epidural is:

a. *De rigueur for a modern labor—only a masochist would forgo one.*

b. *Only for the weak, and a reasonable way to judge what kind of woman you are and mother you'll be.*

c. *A regional anesthetic, administered by an anesthesiologist for the purpose of pain relief during labor or certain surgical procedures.*

(As always, when in doubt, go with "C.")

Both Tracey and Jessica have been my clients. And I can care for them both because I do not have an agenda about how a woman births, other than that her choices are respected and that she feels safe and well supported.

But I do worry a bit about women whose only plan involves getting an epidural. Epidurals are most effective when given in active labor—that is, when contractions are strong, and long, and regular. But it can take many hours for labor to become active, and that time is time best spent at home.

(And no, anesthesiologists do not make house calls.)

Tracey deserves to know that she may need to wait for an epidural; given too early, epidurals can slow the labor process. But there are other ways to cope with pain during labor, both pharmacological and nonpharmacological, and understanding those options may ease her mind. There are risks and benefits to every intervention, and Tracey should also be told the risks and benefits of epidural anesthesia.

I worry, too, about women who are emphatic that they won't need pharmacological pain relief. Usually, labor is progressive. As contractions lengthen and strengthen, the cervix opens and the baby descends. When labor is progressive, if a woman feels safe and well supported, she will generally find that she copes just fine. Almost every woman reaches an "I can't do this" moment, but if she is told, you are doing it, you are so close, she will find the strength to continue.

Sometimes, however, labor is not progressive. And when it's not, the story changes. Effective pain relief can allow a woman to rest, and sometimes, as her pelvis relaxes, the baby rotates and a progressive labor resumes. Sometimes an epidural can help a woman achieve a vaginal delivery.

if a woman feels safe and well supported, she will generally find that she copes just fine

Jessica deserves to know that planning a home birth doesn't guarantee a home birth. She may change her mind and decide she wants pharmacological pain relief in labor, or her midwife might recommend she transfer to the hospital if any risk factors emerge.

While Jessica and Tracey may appear to be polar opposites, they are actually both coming from the same place. And that place is a place of fear. When Tracey says, "I am definitely having an epidural," she may be saying, I am terrified of labor. When Jessica says, "I am absolutely having a home birth," she also may be saying: I am terrified of labor.

Both Tracey and Jessica will benefit from being listened to and supported through their labor—however it unfolds. Both women, that is, will benefit from being treated with kindness and respect—as do we all.

There can be tremendous strength in forgoing an epidural, moving through the raw power of each contraction.

There can be tremendous strength in opting for pain relief, allowing your body to open even as it rests.

So here's another answer for our pop quiz:

d. *An epidural is a safe and effective analgesia that pregnant people in developed countries are lucky enough to be able to access. They may choose an epidural, they may have an indication for an epidural, or they may not want and not need an epidural. Recognizing that having access to safe analgesia is a gift of this particular time and place, let's be grateful for that option rather than judgmental should someone else's choice differ from your own.*

(Was that too long? I knew there was a reason I was never hired to write standardized tests. You get the idea.)

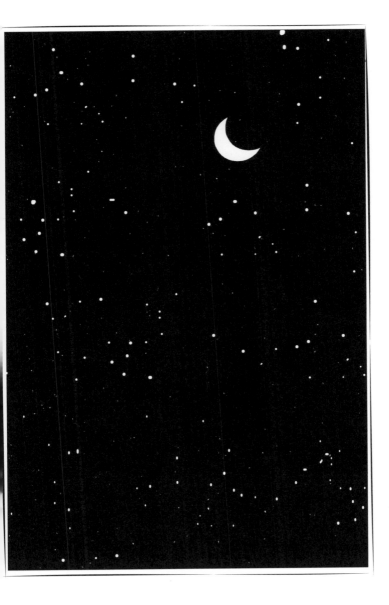

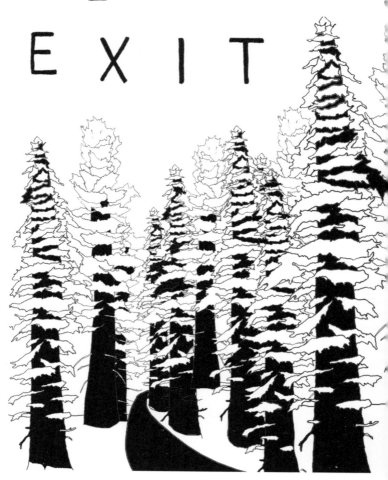

E

IS FOR

EXIT

As a student, I spent a few months working in a community with a large Indigenous population. The midwife there used to quote a saying that one of her clients had taught her. "The elders teach," the midwife would say, "the longer you walk, the shorter your labor."

Walking. It sounds so simple. And yet, it can make such a difference. Not just in labor, but in life. There is more and more research demonstrating that humans were not meant to sit eight hours a day. Our bodies were built to move, and walking benefits our minds and our bodies.

Among maternity care providers, there's a consensus that babies are malpositioned more than they used to be. Midwives talk about "optimal fetal positioning"—trying to get a baby into the best position possible. Ideally, the baby is in an "OA" position—occiput (that's the back of the head) anterior (in front). If you could see inside a woman's pelvis, the OA baby would be facing toward her mother's back, whereas posterior babies (OP) would be looking right back at you. This matters because the presenting diameter (a fancy way of saying: the width of the part that comes first) of an OP baby is just slightly wider than that of an OA baby.

And when it comes to your pelvis—well, every centimeter matters.

There is some evidence that the increase in posterior babies, and the resulting increase in longer, less progressive labors, is a result of our more sedentary lifestyles. If you sit at a desk all day—or if you spend long periods in a car or on public transit—the position of your body (back bowed, stomach sunken) may encourage babies into a posterior position.

And by "some evidence," I mean only that. There aren't any high-quality studies of this phenomenon. To be fair, it'd be a hard study to perform well—there'd be so much to control for, in terms of body type and baby size and labor interventions.

So what's an office-bound gal to do?

Try walking when you can: park a bit farther away, head to the next bus stop, eat your lunch standing up.

When you do sit, try sitting angled slightly forward, with your knees lower than your hips. If you can get hold of one of those birth balls, sit on that. They're wonderful, because they force you to sit up straight, knees wide. If not, tuck a sweatshirt or a small pillow behind you, so that you won't sink back into your desk chair.

At home, try a modified hands-and-knees position

while watching TV: drape yourself over a stack of pillows, or over the birth ball if you have one.

Am I starting to sound insufferable? When I was seven months pregnant with my first child I actually waded into a frigid lake to escape a woman who had ambushed me as I sat with my niece on the beach. "You're pregnant!" she'd announced, as if I hadn't noticed, and then went on to offer me, you guessed it, unsolicited advice. "When labor begins," Anonymous Lake Lady told me, "be sure to scrub the kitchen floor on your hands and knees. Get right down into it—that kind of work helps bring the baby."

I was . . . well, I was appalled. Scrub the kitchen floor on my knees? Really?

That said, after witnessing hundreds of labors, and more malpositioned babies than I'd wish, I now have to admit: if you're gonna hang out a bit on hands and knees, getting a clean kitchen floor out of the process isn't so bad.

A friend of mine who works for a fancy San Francisco–based publisher once described how an ergonomics expert had visited her office, carefully observed everyone at work, and provided individual support—including fancy chair and desk additions, all paid for by her company—to better all of their body mechanics.

If you can get one of those guys to come into your workplace: yes, do that.

If not: remember the wisdom that our client shared. And walk.

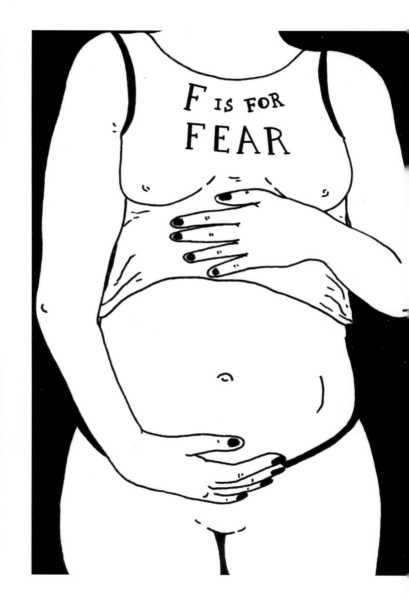

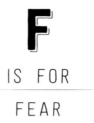

F

IS FOR

FEAR

Midway through my first clinical placement, I assisted at a relatively straightforward delivery that changed the way I thought about birth.

Sarah was a twenty-eight-year-old first-time mom, and she'd had a completely healthy pregnancy. Her water broke at thirty-eight and a half weeks, and contractions began immediately after. By the time Sarah arrived at the hospital she was four to five centimeters dilated, her cervix paper-thin (we call that fully effaced), and her baby nice and low in her pelvis. Within four hours she'd achieved full dilation.

Everything was going so well.

But Sarah refused to push.

I couldn't understand it. When I'd labored with my daughter, the urge to push had been so strong I couldn't hold back. But Sarah curled up, actively resisting. Why wasn't she pushing? What was wrong?

"Push," the midwife said, gentle but firm. "Push—stronger now. Push."

There was no urgency—her baby's heart rate was perfect. Yet Sarah was so resistant that it took a fair amount of active coaching—"knees apart, Sarah, bear down, that's right"—to get her to agree to push at all. If the midwife paused in her encouragement, Sarah would curl up again, shake her head, and say, "No, I can't do it, no."

Most babies have a way of getting themselves born. Despite Sarah's reluctance, she pushed her baby out.

My hands were over the midwife's as we slowly delivered the head: "That's the way, nice and slow." We paused to wait for the next contraction and felt the easy release of the wet body: "Reach on down, Sarah, here's your baby."

The midwife stepped back as I lifted the baby up and into Sarah's arms.

Sarah wrapped her arms tightly around her baby, pressed her lips to his head. The nurse draped warm blankets over him; on cue, he gave a beautiful cry. He curled a hand toward his mouth, wrinkled his forehead.

"He's okay," Sarah repeated, gazing down at her son, "he's okay, he's okay."

Watching Sarah as, sobbing, she kissed her baby, I learned something important. As a student, I'd been focused on birth as a physiological process: embryology, placentation, the stages and phases of labor and delivery. But birth is a psychological journey as well. Everything is at stake, always, and we bring every ounce of ourselves to our children's births.

I'd forgotten—how could I have forgotten?—that

Sarah's older sister had suffered a stillborn baby at thirty-eight weeks. Sarah had supported her sister through tremendous grief and had feared a similar tragedy during her own pregnancy. At her request, the midwife had booked her an obstetric consult for induction at term. Though the obstetrician reminded her that her own pregnancy was low risk, Sarah was adamant: she would be induced by thirty-nine weeks.

When she'd gone into labor spontaneously I'd thought: How wonderful, this is just what she wanted. I hadn't realized how it might feel for Sarah: the final fear of letting go, of pushing her baby out and into the world—the surrender, the terror. And, perhaps also, the guilt that she should have what her sister would not.

Birth is both physiological and psychological. And it is also intensely personal. This is why it matters how we are treated; it matters that we feel safe. At the same time, a difficult labor does not mean that the mother is especially difficult—we're all difficult, after all, in our own ways, and some of us are lucky in labor and some of us aren't.

And almost everyone is afraid.

Acknowledge your fears, if you can, and surround yourself with safety: people who will speak kindly to you, people who will support you.

And then aim straight through the center of that dim tunnel, the length of the narrow bridge.

The only way through is out the other side.

g is for guilt

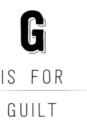

G

IS FOR

GUILT

Be gentle with yourself.

We put a lot of pressure on ourselves: the perfect birth, the perfect baby, the perfect mother.

Know right now that you will not be perfect. You will say and do things you wish you hadn't. More often, you will simply be too distracted or tired or overwhelmed to say or do what you'll wish you would have.

Learn to say "I'm sorry."

But also: learn to be gentle with yourself.

Years ago, I took over for another midwife in the midst of a long birth. Dana had been in labor for many hours and with little change. By the time I came on, she'd received an epidural for rest and Pitocin for labor augmentation, but her baby still didn't seem interested in exiting anytime soon.

We talked about where we were at and the increasing possibility of a cesarean birth.

Dana started to cry. She was scared: not of what the surgery might mean for her but of what it might mean for her baby. She'd read that vaginal birth was better for babies.

"I'm already failing as a mother," Dana said.

Perhaps it was because, at that time, I was so constantly exhausted and overwhelmed by two young children that I answered so quickly, and so bluntly. "Oh gosh," I told her, "don't take this first opportunity to feel guilty. You will have so many better opportunities later on. Let this one go."

Dana looked at me, surprised. Had her midwife really just suggested that she'd have loads of regrets to embrace down the road?

But her own mother, who had been beside her throughout the labor, smiled. "It's true," she said. "You'll have plenty of other chances for guilt. Don't beat yourself up over this."

And then we both told her: You've done your very best.

And she had, and she would.

Be gentle with yourself.

Model the compassion you have for your child by giving that compassion, also, to yourself.

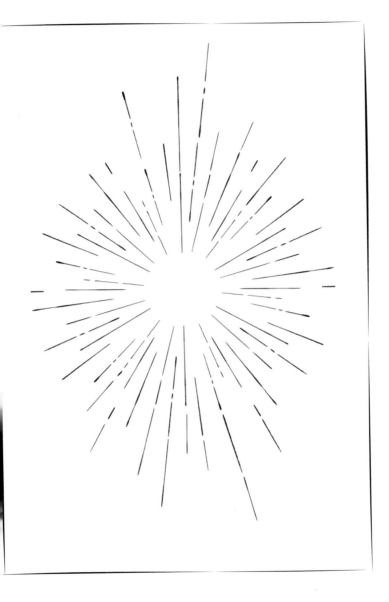

h is for hello

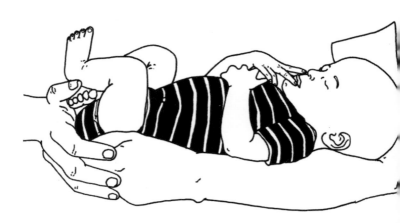

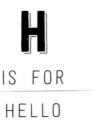

H

IS FOR

HELLO

The moment will come: you will hold your baby.

I was pushing, hard, with my first baby. I was at home, supported by my midwives. And I was hot. "Can we open a window?" I asked.

My midwives said no, the room needed to be warm for the baby.

Something shifted when they said that. The baby, the baby—there was going to be a baby, and her need for warmth was more important than my need for cool air. And I didn't know how to tell my midwives the truth— that it was impossible, wasn't it, that an actual live baby was going to emerge from my vagina? There I was, pushing, and still I thought, I just don't see this happening. But they looked so earnest that I didn't want to disappoint them, and anyway there was another contraction coming, carrying my words away.

And not too much longer, Eva was in my arms.

Hello.

Those first moments with your baby: revel in them. Gaze and gaze and gaze. Laugh and eat and talk, too, but put away your phone, stay off social media, ignore all the beeps and buzzes around you and just take it in, breathe it in. You will not get many moments like this in life.

Bask in that hello. Say it, kiss it, smell it.

Make it last.

"Be present" has become a catchphrase, but if there was ever a time to be present, this is it.

Look and look and look.

Know also: the moment of saying hello may not correspond perfectly with the moment of birth. Sometimes, the room is filled with people and bright lights; sometimes, your baby is rushed away from you. If that happens you may feel helpless, but you are not helpless. Hold space for your baby. Pray if prayer is right for you; tell your baby—out loud, silently, in whatever way feels most true—that you're near.

Eventually, the crowd will clear.

Eventually, your own quiet hello will be heard.

And when that time comes, it will be worth the wait.

A short while after Eva was born, I spoke to my brother, a rabbi, on the phone. At his suggestion, I recited the Shecheyanu, a Jewish blessing of thanks for having been sustained and supported to reach the present moment, or, in the words of the blessing, "this season."

I had never thought that much about the Shecheyanu before—I recited it on cue at holidays, without much reflection. But at that moment, I understood it. I had reached a new season, and I was thankful. As for what would come next—the blessing offered no promises, no assurances. It was just: we have reached this season. We are here, now, and we are grateful.

I said that blessing after the birth of my second child, Tillie, and my third, Avi. I can still conjure the specifics of those moments. The light in the room, the people there with me, even the feel of my newborn in my arms.

All the joy and sorrows in the tomorrows of you and your child's lives remain a wonderful mystery.

But this moment, this season, you can hold forever.

Hello.

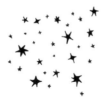

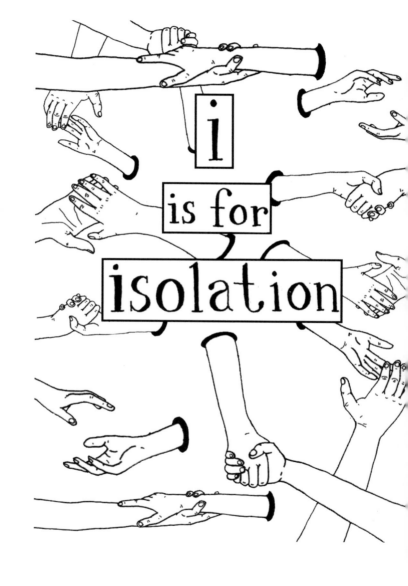

I

IS FOR

ISOLATION

I'm going to talk about the proverbial village again.

There was a time when new mothers would not be left alone with their babies but enveloped, instead, in a maternal sphere of child-rearing. There would have been other young mothers close by for commiseration, and aunts and grandmothers for guidance.

There would have been support.

I recognize that support may not always have been welcome. I know that sometimes it could be restrictive. I know that sometimes it could be abusive.

But parents were not alone.

Many of us, perhaps most of us, have lost community. Many of us, perhaps most of us, feel isolated after birth.

The days can be very long. And very boring.

Creating community is key.

About 90 percent of women experience the "baby blues," a fleeting sadness brought on by the exhaustion and confusion of those early days. After all, most of us are creatures of habit. Becoming a parent is such a major transition, and it can be disorientating and distressing.

The "baby blues" strike early—usually in the first two weeks postpartum. It's a time of upheaval and a time of settling, and it's not a time to make any diagnoses. Just observe, and be kind to yourself.

One of the best pieces of advice I received as a soon-to-be new mother came from a prenatal yoga teacher.

(Not the part when we were told to sit back on our feet with our toes curled underneath us, focusing on and breathing through the pain. That part was just terrible, and all I could think was, This hurts, this hurts, this hurts, and if I can't handle the pain of my toes curled underneath me, then how will I handle labor?

It turns out: they have nothing in common, and I still can't see the purpose of inflicting needless pain on yourself as some kind of labor prep.

But I digress.)

The good advice came at the end of class, when we lay on our mats, just shy of dozing, and our teacher, Sasha, talked. "Every birth is a gift," she said, "but in every birth there is also a loss. And that's the loss of who you were, who your partner was, who you were together, before having a baby." She paused. "It's okay to mourn that loss," she added.

At the time, her words didn't have much meaning for me. I couldn't wait to meet my baby.

A few weeks later, they did.

I did lose myself, a bit, in those early weeks. I did love my baby, but I wasn't always sure I liked her. Everything is topsy-turvy for a little while after a birth: like Alice, you may feel that you've fallen down a rabbit hole.

If you find yourself mourning the life you led, that's okay.

Let yourself feel what you're feeling. Don't be afraid, don't try to shut it down—those feelings are valid, and so very common. Let them come into the light and show you who they are. It may take some time, but once you know these emotions well, know their outlines, their depths, the edges that are smooth and the edges that are ragged, then you will find, too, you know how best to fold them away.

It's a liminal time, a time of transition. It's a time of love and a time of loss.

Postpartum depression, which is more severe than the baby blues, is common enough that it has its own abbreviation: PPD, people say, three letters that roll off the tongue too neatly, belying the anguish of the diagnosis. A better label, as labels go, is PMD: perinatal mood disorders. Perinatal rather than postpartum because these feelings often emerge in pregnancy; mood disorders because a woman may experience depression, anxiety, a combination of both, and even, though rarely, psychosis.

We know that pregnancy and the postpartum period can create a "perfect storm" for depression and anxiety—the disorientation and distress, the insecurity and isolation.

The exhaustion. The hormonal fluctuations.

We also know that the hardest time to reach out can be when a person is most in need.

everything is topsy-turvy for a little while after a birth

If you are reading this while you are pregnant, think about your resources. Have you ever experienced depression or anxiety before? Did anything help you overcome that? Are you experiencing depression or distressing anxiety right now?

(Did those questions just make you totally anxious? I'm sorry. That reaction is normal, of course. But it's still important to ask them.)

(Bear with me while I ask a few more.)

Do you have a therapist? Do you have health-care coverage for a therapist? Can your pregnancy care provider recommend a therapist who takes your insurance?

Do you know other new parents? Are there drop-in groups near you? If not, can you start one?

You have other things to do, I know. But one of the most important things you can do is ensure you have supports in place so that if you need help, you can easily access it. Find out about new parent groups close to you, if you can. Think about things you'd like to do with your baby, after the first few weeks. Identify a therapist or parenting circle, if possible. Ask your care provider who and what they recommend locally.

And if you know another new parent, consider knocking on their door. It's such a particular time and no one knows it quite like those immersed in it. Who else will nod, listening closely, as you recount exactly which hours your baby did and did not sleep the previous night? Who else will understand that cutting a baby's nails is the world's most difficult task and hauling a car seat out of a car and into your home its most draining?

And who knows—that parent may have been waiting desperately for just your knock.

The isolation is real, but it is not inevitable.

A gift you can give yourself: knock on these doors while you're pregnant, so they will already be cracked open when your newborn is in your arms.

J is for

Joy

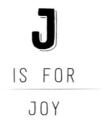

J

IS FOR

JOY

One morning, as I tidied up the living room, I came across one of my daughters' stuffed animals. To be more specific, I came across a blush-pink pony wearing two pairs of girl underwear over her head and a pastel-striped sock on her tail.

I called over my younger daughter, who was around three at the time. I asked something reasonable, like: What's up with this pony?

"Well," my daughter began, "it was a stormy day . . ."

This is the joy of parenting. As an old friend put it, she was perfectly happy with her sepia-toned life before having children. And then she had a son, and her life became Technicolor.

In a sepia world, your living room will not be cluttered with underwear-bedecked ponies.

But nor will your life be so enriched by a child's wild imagination, nor so warmed by baby-chub snuggles.

There's so much focus on everything you can't do with a baby.

Like: eat a meal while it's hot, without interruption.

Or sleep through the night.

Or—but wait, I was taking another tack here.

Because here's the thing: there's so much you can do with a baby, with a child, that you couldn't or wouldn't do without one.

sing your

baby

to sleep

I learned this lesson when our oldest was less than a week old. My husband and I are both tone-deaf—no one ever wants to hear us sing. Yet when my husband sang to our daughter, rocking her gently as he walked slow circles around our bedroom, she fell asleep.

He looked at me, full of wonder. "I've never sung anyone to sleep before!"

Sing your baby to sleep. Snuggle him when he wakes. Spy on her as she plays with some toys, illuminated by a ray of sunlight coming through the kitchen window. Kiss his finger where it hurts, and marvel at how your kisses can comfort.

Gather in the joy. There will be so much joy, and it's there for the taking.

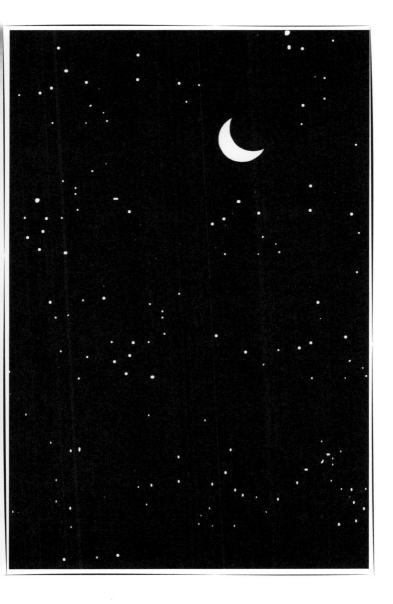

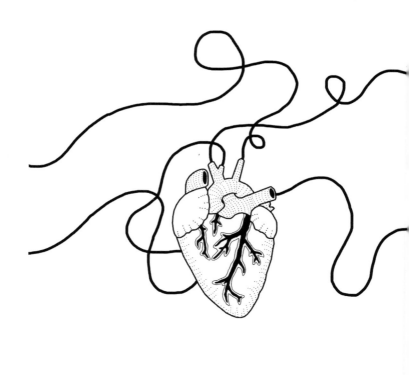

K is for Kick

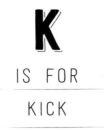

K

IS FOR

KICK

Early in pregnancy, most of us long for that first kick. The weeks go so slowly—have weeks ever gone so slowly before? Suddenly you're tracking Wednesdays, or whatever day it was that you've established as the first day of your last menstrual period, counting them on your fingers, crossing them off the calendar, listening for the chime as your pregnancy-tracker phone app announces a new week begun.

Then your baby is born and you keep counting weeks, though now it's the birthing day you track. One Tuesday, two Tuesdays, three.

Eventually you'll move to months. You'll forget about the day of the week, and follow the date of birth instead.

Four months, five.

After the fastest-slowest time you can remember, you'll be rounding up: "almost a year," you'll tell someone, and smile as your four-toothed baby waves hello.

Then a year and a half. And now you don't notice the birth date pass each month anymore—you're focused on two, then three, then four.

As they say: the days are long, but the years are short.

But nothing is as long as those first few weeks of pregnancy. Those exist, for most of us, in their own universe of molasses-slow time. First-time parents typically feel that first kick around nineteen or twenty weeks—if you're reading this in the first trimester, that may seem like an impossibly long wait.

Somehow the time passes, as time always does.

And hopefully as it does you'll be rewarded with the very thing you've longed for: a kick.

At first it's vague: Was that a kick? Could it have been?

Then eventually, it's unmistakable—there it is, again.

It may feel uncomfortable at times. It may be surprisingly inconvenient. It may seem strangely cognizant—like the time my third baby kicked my second child squarely in the head as she rested against my belly.

But if you think about it—well, it's one of the more incredible things you're likely to experience in a lifetime.

If you're reading this while pregnant: inside you, a tiny heart is beating. Organs are forming. Eyelashes are thickening. And a little leg or arm may be reaching out, right at this moment, to test the limits of its known world.

the days are long, but the years are short

And when it does: what a marvelous event.

Before we see our babies or smell them, touch them or hear them, they touch us.

It's a metaphor, maybe, for parenting. Because as much as we all strive to raise our children well, ultimately, where they lead, we will follow.

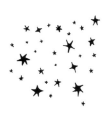

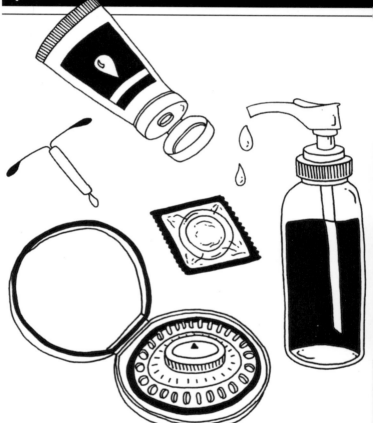

L IS FOR LUBRICANT

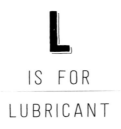

IS FOR

LUBRICANT

Every now and then women ask me if it's definitely positively absolutely safe to have sex during pregnancy.

The answer is: yes, usually.

To clarify: in certain situations, we advise clients not to have sex—if a placenta is very close to the cervix, for instance, or if there is a particular threat of preterm labor.

Most of the time, however, sex is perfectly healthy in pregnancy. More than that: as your body changes, it can be affirming and exciting to feel desire and to be met with desire.

"What gets the baby in gets the baby out," I was taught by an experienced midwife, and there's definitely some truth to the old adage. If your partner is biologically male: sperm contains prostaglandins, which help ripen the cervix at term, when receptors for those prostaglandins appear on the cervix. But there's no need to feel left out if your partner doesn't have a penis or if you're parenting solo: the female orgasm releases oxytocin, the same hormone that causes uterine contractions. That's what an orgasm is, actually—a series of contractions. And while an orgasm likely won't launch you into labor, certainly sex can help ready your body for the journey.

So far, so good. Sex during pregnancy is almost always safe, and sex can help bring on labor. And then labor begins. And then you have a baby. And then . . .

And then the story changes.

In my practice, I always ask about contraception at the one-month postpartum visit. "What's your plan?" I ask, reminding my clients that while breastfeeding makes pregnancy unlikely, it's far from a guaranteed method of birth control.

The vast majority of women look at me with bleary eyes and say something like, "Abstinence? Forever?"

Take the time you need. And it will take at least some time: for your body to heal, for your hormones to settle, for you to remember your sexual self and emerge from exhaustion long enough to think, yeah, I'm ready to feel that way again.

And when that happens you'll need two things:

One, patience from your partner, if you have one.

And, two, a good water-based lubricant.

Yes, this is one of those situations where a particular product really can make a difference. One of the more interesting studies I've ever read looked at discomfort during sex at three months postpartum. The conclusion? Women who had cesarean sections reported the same level of discomfort during sex as women who'd had vaginal births.

It's obvious why sex would feel uncomfortable soon after vaginal birth, but why would a cesarean delivery affect vaginal sensation?

There's a simple answer. Breastfeeding suppresses estrogen, which is the hormone responsible for vaginal lubricant. Without that lubricant, sex is dry. And if it's dry, it's uncomfortable.

This makes sense from an evolutionary perspective. For millennia, a woman and her baby's best chance of survival depended on pregnancy spacing. We literally don't go into heat when we're taking care of a newborn.

Modern times, however, sometimes call for evolutionary work-arounds. And luckily this work-around can be purchased at just about any gas station.

So, when it comes to resuming sex after pregnancy, move slowly and invest in a good lube.

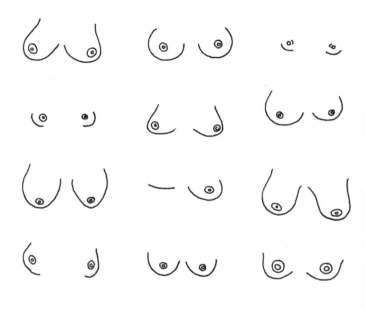

M IS FOR **MILK**

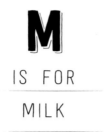

M

IS FOR

MILK

Before pregnancy, breasts have a fairly singular role in our culture. They're sex symbols.

And yet, once the baby comes, they have a new job. Food production.

When I was pregnant, I puzzled over this. I imagined my breasts as some vain, narcissistic woman, hitherto concerned only with appearance, suddenly announcing a newfound passion for solving world hunger.

You'd roll your eyes. You'd think, yeah, right.

And yet: most breasts do make that transition. They announce a career change, and, voilà, they've moved from modeling to making milk.

After all: we are mammals, and this is what mammals do. In fact, it's what defines our class.

(That's not to say it has to define you.)

As a midwife, I have supported hundreds of pregnant people through the early days and weeks of breastfeeding. And having done so, I will be the first to say: very few find it easy at first.

After pregnancy, after labor, and delivery, it would be nice if the breastfeeding part would just come naturally, wouldn't it?

It would be. But don't bet on it.

Most new parents have a few challenges setting out. Women receive scant postpartum care: the obstetrician hands us off to the pediatrician, and neither specialist provides breastfeeding support. Most of our own mothers formula-fed; we may not have seen a lot of breastfeeding mamas, and we may not have a close friend or relative to help us. We're also just plain exhausted after giving birth, and it's difficult to master yet another skill when you're so very tired.

The first few days you worry because your baby is losing weight. Perhaps a few people have already questioned whether "he's getting enough," and though you've been told that your baby's belly is the size of a pea and that colostrum is rich with antibodies, it sometimes takes twenty minutes to latch her and your nipples are raw and, really, is it worth it?

And then your milk comes in. And your breasts are

full and aching, and the veins are dark and puffy under your skin, and it feels like your body will never just be your body again, and the baby won't sleep, and your nipples are still raw, and you're certain that the last feed just ended so how can it already be time for the next one to begin?

And you read, somewhere, that it wasn't supposed to hurt.

But it hurts.

And maybe the baby won't latch well, or maybe she won't let up. Maybe you have to wake him from a deep sleep to try to feed, or maybe he wakes abruptly every time you try to lay him down.

Every experience is different, but for most parents, breastfeeding is an uphill battle.

You may wonder: Can this possibly be worth it?

I would say: yes.

But you may need some support.

It is absolutely not necessary to breastfeed to be a good parent. But once you and your baby get the hang of it, breastfeeding does make life easy. You make food for your baby. It's always ready, it's always the right temperature, and it's free. There's nothing to buy or clean or prepare or worry about accidentally leaving at home.

You are the food.

A trick that helped me during those awkward, early

days: I reminded myself that there were selfish reasons to breastfeed, too.

Women who breastfeed have lower rates of breast and ovarian cancer.

Women who breastfeed also report lower rates of depression postpartum.

But the flip side of that last fact: women who wanted to breastfeed but don't succeed report increased depression.

Try not to judge yourself in these early days. Remember that there are so many ways to be a good mother, and that formula is food for your baby, too. If you want to breastfeed, plan for it just a bit. Try to find someone who can help you, in case you need help. Maybe it's another new mom, or a relative, or a friend's relative, or a lactation consultant, or a nurse, or a La Leche League member, or your clinical care provider.

remember that there are so many ways to be a good mother

Whoever it is: get that number now, so that you won't have to go searching later.

Most of the time all you need is a little help with positioning and some old-fashioned encouragement.

Sometimes more help is needed. And sometimes the

baby is losing just too much weight despite all efforts, and expressed breast milk or donated breast milk or formula is needed to keep your baby on track.

That's okay too. We are lucky to be able to provide good food for our babies, in whatever way is best.

I have a hard time believing in the much-publicized formula versus breastfeeding wars. Perhaps there really are legions of women making others feel terrible for their feeding choices, but I suspect we are blaming women for what is actually a societal failure: a lack of support, including hands-on assistance for establishing breast-feeding and time off from work to maintain it, for new mothers.

Please don't judge yourself for how easy or hard this is for you. If you want to breastfeed but are struggling to do so, imagine your child full-grown. Imagine your daughter struggling to breastfeed her child, or your son or daughter struggling to support a partner through her own breast-feeding difficulties. Think about the message you'd want to send. Think about how you'd console that struggling mother, remind her of all the ways she's wonderful, tell her how lucky her baby is just to be so loved.

If you need to, tell that to yourself. Over and over and over.

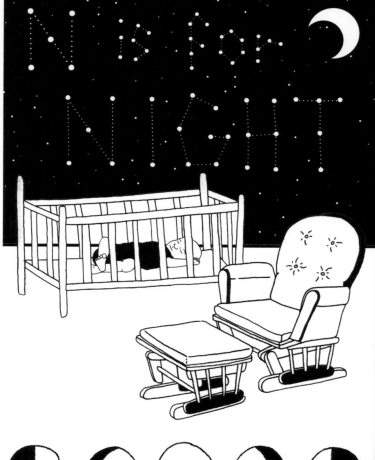

N

IS FOR

NIGHTS WITH
A NEWBORN

"She falls asleep when I'm holding her," Laura tells me, her voice pressured. There is something important she needs me to understand. "But then, as soon as I lay her down—she wakes up!"

I nod. I've heard this one before.

We've all been tricked. As children, we were given dolls. When we laid them down, their lashed eyelids closed; when we picked them up, they opened wide in blue-plastic wonder.

Real babies, it turns out, are the exact opposite. Rock them in your arms and those lovely eyelids close; lay them down and voilà, their eyes (and their mouths) fly open.

And who can blame them? Your baby spent nine months growing inside you and continues to crave warmth and touch and movement.

As a new mom, I was woefully unprepared for this. Our midwife told us that two or three hours should pass from the start of one feed to the start of the next, but that in a twenty-four-hour period our baby could have one (but not more than one) five-hour break. My husband and I actually debated whether this longer break would be better scheduled between midnight and five a.m. or one a.m. to six a.m. Which would leave us best rested, we wondered?

What were we thinking?

There was no five-hour break that night, of course. It hardly seemed like there was any break at all. She fed, she fell asleep, I laid her down, she woke up. And repeat.

So what's an exhausted new parent to do?

Don't get too excited—I don't have an easy answer.

But here's something. First: familiarize yourself with safe sleep recommendations. Your baby is safest on his own surface in your bedroom, free of any blankets, pillows, or soft bedding accessories.

This is all the more important if you smoke, even if no one smokes inside the house.

(Please don't let anyone smoke inside your house.)

Ask around: everyone has a trick for helping a baby sleep. Some parents swear by the mom's shirt as a bottom sheet, or a hot water bottle to warm the bassinet, or a swaddle-style sleep sac.

Whatever trick you try—and doubtless you will try many—be careful that it doesn't compromise sleep safety. A shirt tightly tucked into the mattress is fine; loose bedding is not. A warmed mattress might help—but don't forget to remove the heat source before placing the baby down, as overheating increases sudden infant death syndrome (SIDS) risk.

Here's the thing: little by little, your baby will sleep longer and longer. What didn't work one night may well work the next: don't give up on that bassinet just yet. But going it alone will be hard in the early days—if you don't have a partner, see if anyone can come stay with you to spell you during the nights. And if you do have a partner, make sure your partner is on board for helping, too.

Eventually, when your baby is a few months old, you might decide to try a sleep-training approach. And here's a warning: if you want to watch a group of adults completely lose their minds, ask about sleep training.

It's like throwing a squirrel into a piranha pond.

And, no, I don't really know anything about squirrel-piranha interactions. But I do know that parents can be passionate on the topic of sleep training. And by passionate I mean, terribly judgmental, with some swearing that you're crazy if you don't do it, and others arguing that you're criminal if you do.

As with everything: trust yourself. Remember that your baby is not everyone's baby, and your needs may be different from someone else's. Remember, too, that ultimately we need to care for ourselves if we are to care for our babies.

Long nights will pass, I promise. And, far-fetched as it may seem now, one day you might just miss watching the sun rise while cradling your baby.

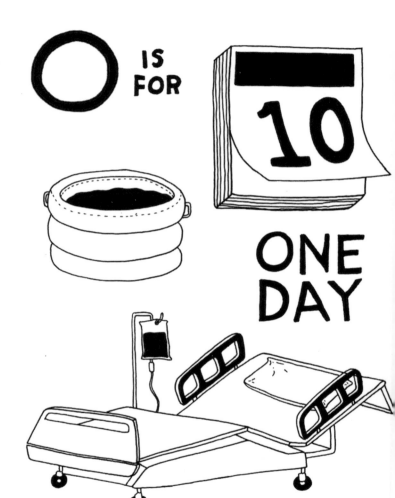

O IS FOR

10

ONE DAY

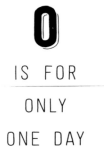

IS FOR

ONLY

ONE DAY

Some people say, birth is only one day. As in: it doesn't matter all that much, ultimately.

Clearly, I am not one of those people.

Ask the oldest woman you know to tell you about her child's birth. She will remember; she will have a story.

It is not just one day—not for her, not even after all these years.

Birth matters.

Every time a woman advocates for the birth she wants, someone will say something like, you're prioritizing your experience over your baby's safety.

Maybe such a person exists . . . somewhere. But I have never met her. I have never met a woman who placed anything before her baby's safety.

Never.

But women have different ideas of safety.

For most people, safety is birthing at a hospital. This has been the community standard for a few generations. You were probably born in a hospital, and your parents and grandparents were likely born in hospitals too. And in this time of birthing at hospitals, birth has become so much safer. We have standard training now: excellent doctors and nurses and midwives who have studied for years to be able to attend women in labor. We have antibiotics, and access to blood products, and evidence-based medicine.

grieving for the birth you didn't have doesn't make you a bad mother, it makes you human

We have so much to be so grateful for.

Some women may plan to give birth at a birthing center or at home. Those women are likely aware of excellent research that demonstrates that, for low-risk women attended by midwives, out-of-hospital birth is as safe as hospital birth. There are variables in play, including what constitutes low-risk, what the transfer protocol would be should a complication arise, and what training your care provider has.

In Canada, where I work, all Registered Midwives must maintain both home and hospital privileges. All our clients, even those planning home birth, register at the local hospital; if a client wants to transfer to the hospital during labor, or if we recommend she does so, we can continue to manage her labor at the hospital just as we did at home—the transfer process is smooth because home birth is fully integrated into the maternity system.

Wherever you plan to give birth, and wherever you end up giving birth, I can guarantee you one thing: the story will matter.

It may be a source of pride, a story of joy, one you love to tell.

It may be disappointing, difficult, even deeply upsetting.

If you find yourself grieving over the birth you didn't have, let yourself have those feelings. People will say, "All that matters is a healthy baby." But as childbirth educator and doula Penny Simkin has written, the woman's experience matters, too.

Grieving for the birth you didn't have doesn't make you a bad mother; it makes you human.

Any society that values women should value how women are treated in birth.

Any care provider who values women should devote herself to treating women with compassion and respect.

Whatever happens, it will be more than just one day for you.

P IS FOR

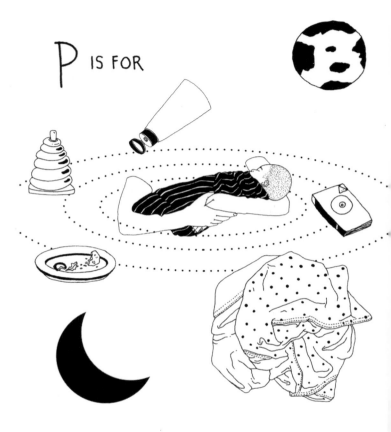

PLANET NEWBØRN

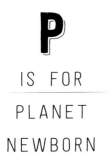

P

IS FOR

PLANET

NEWBORN

In obstetrics we talk about the 4 Ps: the passage and the passenger, the power of contractions, and the position of the baby.

Together, those Ps determine whether the labor will be progressive or not.

I'm not going to write about those 4 Ps, but a fifth.

Planet Newborn.

What is Planet Newborn? Planet Newborn is a place that looks a lot like Earth. Your earth. For instance, your bedroom on Planet Newborn will look almost identical to your bedroom at home, but the discerning eye will be able to pick out small differences. Perhaps there's a small tube of Lansinoh nipple cream on the bedside table. Ditto a plate of unfinished food. A hand towel on the mattress will cover a spot where the baby's diaper leaked—you're going to change the sheets, but you haven't had a chance yet. Maybe there's a book about breastfeeding in the corner of the room—lying right where you hurled it last night. There's a bassinet against the wall that looks perfectly clean—perhaps because your baby has thus far refused to sleep in it.

In the living room lies a heap of bright, plastic, battery-operated toys—exactly the kind you swore you weren't going to get. Who bought them? When did they get here? Why does it take thirty minutes to leave the house? Why, when your partner walked out the door this morning, did you feel so abandoned, so broken, so sure you would never walk out a door with such clarity and confidence again?

You're tired on Planet Newborn. So, so tired. The days are long; the nights are longer. Showering feels like a spa.

You won't be sure about Planet Newborn. You might think: I wish I hadn't come. You might think: This isn't what I signed up for. You might think: Help.

That's okay. That's all normal. Because here's the thing about Planet Newborn: you won't be staying long.

When you started this journey, you thought you were going to have a baby. The kind that smiles and coos and giggles. The kind that makes eye contact.

But it's not a baby that you birth. No: the baby comes later. At birth, you get a newborn.

Newborns are fascinating in an alien-creature way. They have that wise old-man look, they're soft and warm and they smell delicious. If you've had one before, then you know how special they are, and also how fleeting your time with this creature will be.

So if you find yourself feeling lost, just remember: This is Planet Newborn. You will not live here long. Soon, you will return to Earth. And when you do, it'll be even better than before. Because you'll have this wonderful baby beside you.

(And if you're one of those rare birds who skips Planet Newborn entirely and somehow goes straight to Planet Baby Bliss—do yourself a favor if you want to keep those new parent friends and don't gloat.)

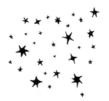

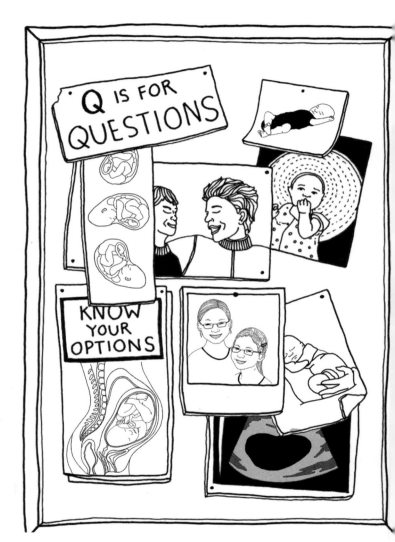

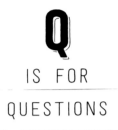

IS FOR

QUESTIONS

Natalie and Tim look at me expectantly. I have just outlined the genetic testing options offered in our province: what the testing looks for, when it's offered, and what a positive result might mean. They sit side by side, facing a bulletin board filled with baby photos. Just a few minutes before, they'd been pointing to a baby they recognized, making note of an appealing name on an official announcement. But that was before I outlined private versus public testing options, quoted the risk of a chromosomal abnormality for women in Natalie's age range. They glance at each other, and then back at me.

"What do most people do?" Natalie asks me. "What do you recommend?"

They would like me to tell them: do this, then this.

But I won't.

It's not that I want to hold out on Natalie and Tim. I understand the desire to be told: here's the right answer, choose this one. But pregnancy is personal, and there isn't one right answer for everyone.

Informed choice is a tenet of midwifery. We recognize the pregnant person as the primary decision maker. As I tell clients: it's your body, and it's your baby, and therefore you (perhaps along with your partner) are the best person to make decisions for your pregnancy.

As a care provider, my job is to ensure that my clients know what options are available, what the evidence says, what risks and benefits a given test or procedure might entail, what the community standard is, and what, if any, recommendation I might have based on their particular clinical picture. In other words, the "informed" part of "informed choice" is on me.

From there, my job is to respect and support their choices.

"It's your choice," I tell Natalie and Tim. "Just as you'll make decisions for your child, so you make decisions in pregnancy."

And a lot of people may have a lot of judgment about those decisions.

But ultimately you decide what feels right for your family.

And that's what parenting is.

Natalie turns to Tim. They begin to talk, together, about how they feel about genetic testing and what they might decide to do if they had a positive result. I remind them that they have time to think about it, and we make a plan for a follow-up meeting. But already their choices are becoming informed, not just by the statistics I provided, but also by their own values: this is what matters to us, now.

Pregnancy should not feel like a checklist: first do this, then this, then this. It is not a one-size-fits-all kind of experience. Don't be afraid to ask questions of your care provider: What will this bloodwork look for? What might this ultrasound tell us? If your care provider seems put out to have to explain routine testing, see if you can find someone else: none of this is routine for you, after all.

One of the joys of my work is seeing families return in subsequent pregnancies, the newborn I last saw at six weeks of age now an active toddler crunching Goldfish on the clinic couch, angling to remove the stethoscope from my hands. In another pregnancy, Natalie and Tim might remember what they chose the first time around, and they might make the same choice again. But just as often clients explain, "Last time I did that, but this time . . ."

Take pleasure in the experience of making decisions, for the very first time, for your child. Ask questions of your care provider and of friends and family you trust. Seek out wisdom—and trust yourself, too.

Parenting begins in pregnancy.

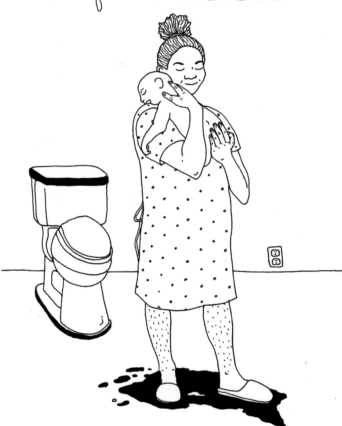

r is for resilience

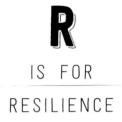

R

IS FOR

RESILIENCE

Several years ago, a client of mine, Lucy, gave birth awfully close to the toilet. She was at the hospital having her second baby; things changed fast, she called out for me, and in the end she delivered standing up in our tiny hospital bathroom. I crouched beside her and caught her baby; she reached down and brought her baby to her chest. A nurse rushed in to help and together we eased Lucy and her baby into bed. When I think of Lucy's birth, I remember her standing tall under the bright bathroom lights, cradling her new baby in shock and delight.

A few hours after the birth, I took Lucy over to the postpartum unit. I helped the nurses settle her and her daughter and then gave her nurse "report"—a brief summary of mom and babe. "The baby came quickly in the end," I mentioned. "She delivered in the bathroom—I wasn't expecting it."

As I walked away, I overheard the nurse calling out, as she returned to Lucy's room, "I heard you had a traumatic birth."

It actually stopped me in my tracks. I hadn't said traumatic. Lucy certainly hadn't said traumatic. Why had she?

The next morning, one of the first questions Lucy asked was, "That delivery—was that traumatic?"

Resilience has become a catchword in recent years. People talk about building resilience, particularly in children. The idea is to help children achieve some kind of solid inner strength that will help them surmount obstacles in life.

Some of us are more resilient than others. We don't get dealt equal decks in life, and it's true, too, that the same experience may be incredibly stressful and negative (even traumatic) to one person but not to another.

There's no easy recipe to build resilience, but there's some evidence to show that people who notice the positive aspects of even the most difficult experiences are more resilient: they weather stress more easily and recover more quickly. I have been amazed by clients who have wept as they recount a difficult miscarriage but then say something like, "One good thing—it did bring me and my partner closer." Those who identify as belonging to a community are also more likely to exhibit resilience: recovery is easier when we are supported, when we are heard and met with love.

Labor & Delivery is generally the happiest of hospital wings—except when it isn't. A traumatic event on L&D is all the more traumatic because it is a place of tremendous hope and fierce love, a place for beginnings rather than endings.

In an ideal world, we would never know if we were resilient. We would never be tested.

In the real world, you may have a strong sense of how well you cope with stress, of whether you ruminate on negative thoughts or tend to focus on positive events.

I don't mean to suggest that a traumatic birth can or should be mitigated by "positive thoughts" along a clichéd everything-happens-for-a-reason continuum.

Sometimes there is no reason. Sometimes there are tragedies.

More often, however, experiences can be viewed through different lenses depending on who does the viewing and what we ourselves bring to it. And while as a care provider I may be asked to help frame an event for a client—"When did this happen? What were you thinking then?"—it is not my place to classify a woman's experience.

Lucy and I talked through her birth. "Was it traumatic for you?" I asked her.

She thought about it, reflecting aloud about the surprising and overwhelming pressure she'd felt to push. She apologized for the mess (women always apologize for the mess) and remembered the strange stunted-walk back to the bed, her babe in her arms, the umbilical cord still linked to her placenta.

"Still," she told me, smiling. "It was kind of awesome."

I wish this for all pregnant people: birth that has a clear kind of awesome.

S is for Serendipity

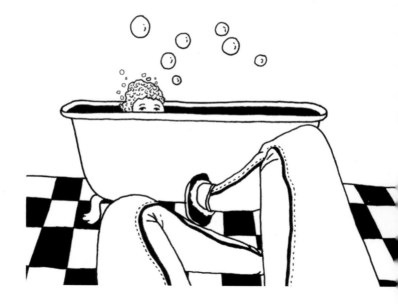

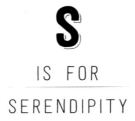

IS FOR

SERENDIPITY

Serendipity is one of those wonderful words that makes you happy (and by you, maybe I mean just me, but I hope I mean you, too) to say aloud.

Just like its meaning: an unexpected treasure found while searching for something else.

Parenting is filled with serendipities. In no small part because sometimes, one of the challenges of parenting can be that we expect to enjoy it.

We take our child to the zoo, and we want the trip to match an image in our minds: a child holding a balloon with one hand and our hand with the other, gazing with wonder at, say, monkeys playing.

And the reality is: your child has a meltdown in the ticket line. The balloons cost $15, so you try to keep her from even noticing them, but she does, so you tell her "maybe later," and yank her toward the monkeys, then watch in horror as a monkey dismembers a pigeon while your child watches. You spent $30 on food your child barely eats and can't find the car on the way out. The much-anticipated outing is a disaster; you need a day off after your day off.

But then: you pour bubbles in the bath, and she spends forty-five minutes playing with a boat and a Tupperware container while you read a novel beside the tub, keeping her company, and every now and then you look up and her face is shining with delight.

Often, the finest moments are those we don't orchestrate.

We live in a time when we are bombarded with images of other people, other families, seemingly enjoying life more than we are. In their photos, everyone is smiling and looking at the camera. In their posts, their children are always making clever comments and bringing home perfect report cards. They are better-looking and more successful, their kitchens are cleaner, their cars undented.

We're all pressed up to the proverbial glass, gazing at what others have and feeling inadequate.

But then again: they're pressed up against the same glass, peering with envy at someone else (or maybe even back at you—you did post that one impressive zoo photo, after all).

A holiday outing can be fantastic, but it's the every-dayness that you'll look back on with nostalgia and long-ing. The pleasure of ordinary moments: reading together on the couch, kneeling down to examine a curious bug beside the schoolyard, singing the same old song at bed-time, arranging the covers just so, kissing good night.

Try to notice these serendipitous moments, the unex-pected treasures in an ordinary day. Listen closely to your children's high, clear voices; the easy giggles and off-key tunes.

Often, the finest moments are those we don't orchestrate

Because here's another special word, and one I never really under-stood before I became a parent: bit-tersweet.

I knew bittersweet, truly and for the first time, when I folded away my daughter's newborn clothes and tucked them into a storage bin. Although I was pleased and proud to be moving-on-up to three-to-six-month-size clothing, I was also just a little heartbroken to think that she would never wear that aqua polka-dotted onesie again, or those tiny cat-face leggings.

Watching a child grow is so deliciously bittersweet.

Savor all the serendipities along the way.

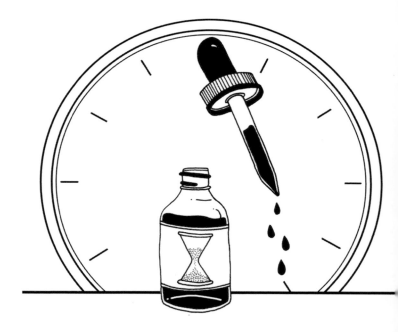

T IS
FOR

IS

TIME

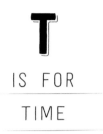

T

IS FOR

TIME

Birth tends to begin at night.

Not always. Not for everyone. But for most of us.

It must have served some evolutionary purpose once. Women are so vulnerable during labor—if danger came, how could they flee? Darkness protected them, kept them hidden under the cloak of night.

Care providers teach most clients not to page them too soon. That's because the evidence is clear—for a low-risk pregnancy, the longer you labor on your own, in your own space, the less likely you are to have unnecessary interventions that do not improve outcomes.

Yes, even if you have a midwife.

Back in the 1950s, Dr. Emanuel Friedman, an obstetrician, observed the length of labor of five hundred white women birthing at a single hospital, then plotted their dilation, by centimeter, on a graph. For the next several decades, the "Friedman curve," as it came to be known, became gospel for what "normal" dilation over time should look like.

Many things have changed since the 1950s, including that first-time moms tend to be older and babies tend to be larger, and for both of those reasons labor may be longer than the norm (and a very limited idea of "the norm") sixty years ago. Recognizing this, the American College of Obstetricians and Gynecologists (ACOG) and the Society for Maternal-Fetal Medicine (SMFM) issued a 2014 consensus statement that said, among other things, that the Friedman curve should no longer be used to define normal labor progress.

time is one of the best things we can give a laboring woman

The reason why all this matters so much is that in the U.S., half of all primary cesarean sections are performed for "failure to progress." By redefining how we measure labor progress, we can reduce that primary cesarean section rate. For instance, new guidelines state that first-time moms should not even be considered to be in active labor (and therefore held up to labor progress standards) until they are six centimeters dilated—whereas the Friedman curve began at three centimeters.

So back to early labor, in your own home.

Unless there is a medical reason to come to the hospital—there are many medical reasons to come to the hospital, and your care provider will inform you about them—it makes sense to wait until you are in a really solid, active labor pattern before leaving home.

Sounds straightforward, right?

And yet, most of the time, when that first contraction hits . . .

People forget it all.

There's a mixture of excitement and panic, and a rush of adrenaline. The partner begins timing the contractions ("Are you feeling one now? Has it ended? Has a new one begun?"). The woman quickly moves through all the positions she's read about: on the ball/on her side/on hands and knees/in the bath.

And in this way, everyone is exhausted before active labor has really begun.

A wise midwife once told me: "Every woman fears the pain of labor, but the enemy in labor isn't pain, it's exhaustion."

Try to rest during early labor. Breathe through that panic, swallow the excitement.

Wait.

Eventually, the contractions will tighten into a pattern, and you will find yourself in a different space. It gets harder but also easier. The uncertainty of early labor is often the most challenging part of the entire process; once labor is active, you are where you have been wanting to go.

(Even if you desperately wish you weren't going there anymore—don't worry, that's normal, too.)

Years ago, I sat with a laboring woman through a golden autumn day. In the beginning, everything went well. I crouched beside her as she leaned over a birth ball during a contraction, moaning softly, and I thought, *This is exactly what she wanted*, and I felt proud to be helping her have the birth I knew she'd hoped for.

And then time passed, and, rather than dilate, her cervix began to swell. I felt terrible telling her that things were not as fantastically progressive as we'd been hoping, and I told her, too, that I would be consulting the obstetrician. But he was busy with several other deliveries, and because my client and her baby were perfectly stable, we supported her to rest and wait for his assessment. And when he came—and introduced himself and obtained her consent to examine her—he smiled and said, "The baby has come down, the head has rotated beautifully, your cervix is no longer swollen, and everything looks great."

And turning to me he said, "You know what that is? The tincture of time."

Time is one of the best things we can give a laboring woman. Not only that: it's what you and your baby deserve. Choose your support people wisely, and rest during early labor, and don't be afraid to ask, of yourself and of others, "Is it time? Do we have more time?"

Take that tincture.

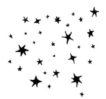

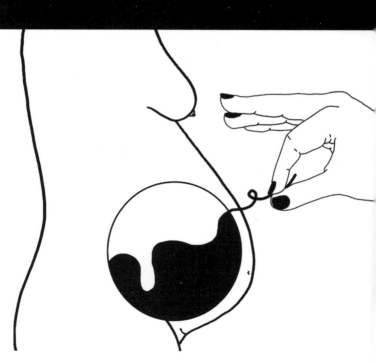

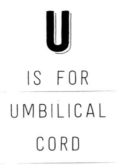

U

IS FOR

UMBILICAL

CORD

The research is clear: there is benefit to delayed cord clamping, which means waiting for the umbilical cord to stop pulsing (and therefore to stop delivering blood to the baby) before clamping and cutting it.

While it's nice to have the evidence, it's strange, in a way, that we needed it. Why would we think cutting the cord instantly conferred benefit? It fits into a pattern of messing with stuff that doesn't need to be messed with: cutting the cord to bring the baby to a warmer to suction her (why?) and measure her (is that necessary to do right away?) and clean her (really?) before finally returning a stunned and stunningly wrapped baby to her mother, who is herself a much more perfect newborn warmer than anything we might cook up.

That's not to say that there's never a reason to cut the cord sooner rather than later. It's just that immediate clamping and cutting should be the exception, not the norm—particularly as the protocol for newborn resuscitation begins with thirty seconds of vigorous stimulation, a task that is easily, and more effectively, accomplished with the cord intact.

But here's the other thing about umbilical cords: no matter when it is cut, in a way it will never be severed.

Not for you.

The cord stops pulsing. It is clamped, it is cut. The mother lifts her newborn higher on her chest, gazes into her eyes. But though their bodies are separated, in those early years the parent's body is still an extension of the child's. The love flows so freely between them. Time will pass, and the child will grow; in growing up there is a growing apart, growing from an intertwined love with few boundaries to an adult love, an independent love.

And we want that for our children.

But that doesn't mean it's easy to let go.

The evidence says: wait at least one minute before clamping and cutting the cord unless there's a good reason to intervene sooner.

The heart says: that cord remains connected forever.

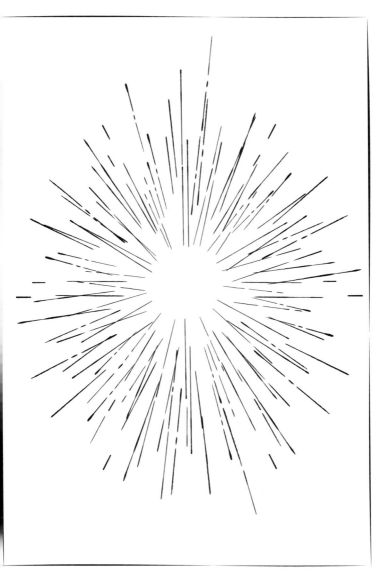

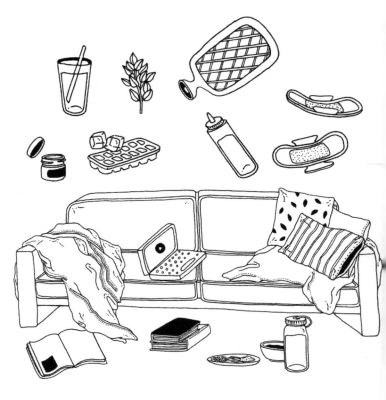

IS FOR VICRYL

V

IS FOR

VICRYL

Vicryl: a strong, synthetic, self-dissolving suture.

Let's talk about tearing. (Did you just cross your legs?)

Midwives do everything we can to prevent tearing. There's no one-size-fits-all approach, but your midwife might use warm compresses or oil or lubricant to help your perineum stretch, and, assuming your baby's heart rate is lovely as can be, she will definitely coach you through a nice, slow delivery of the head and shoulders.

(Are you wondering what a perineum is and whether you even have one? Don't worry: you're not alone. The perineum is the area between the vagina and the anus. Author-midwife Ina May Gaskin famously dubbed it the "taint": "'taint what's above and 'taint what's below.")

Yet sometimes, even when we do everything we can to prevent tearing, women tear. And there are two important things you need to know about this.

First, at almost every birth, the woman will ask me, just after gasping and greeting and kissing her baby, "Did I tear?" That's right: women always ask, because they don't know. Epidural or not, there's so much pressure at the moments before and during birth that you don't actu-ally feel a perineal tear happening.

Isn't that reassuring, in an I-never-thought-that-would-be-reassuring way?

Second, when you see, as I have, lots of women tear and lots of women heal, you realize that we are meant to open and to close again. It's not that tearing is inevitable, at all. But the vagina and perineum are mucous membrane, an incredibly elastic, resilient area that heals beautifully. Our bodies open for birth, and, though it may seem impossible in the first days following, they close again, too.

A cesarean section incision is different—you will be left with a surgical scar. It will be very low and, as a result, private, and as the years pass it will fade until it is almost imperceptible. But it will never disappear. And would you want it to? Among the bravest of scars is that marking the woman who lay down on the stainless-steel table and birthed into the bright lights of the OR.

There are all sorts of recipes to promote perineal heal-ing, and in recent years upscale baby stores have started stocking expensive herbal blends for the bath. While those make wonderful gifts, your perineum is actually a pretty cheap date.

You'll really just need two things: water and rest.

Water: to drink, to place frozen against your perineum, to bathe in if you have a bath and to squirt from a squirt bottle while you urinate (so it won't burn). You can even make your own frozen pads in advance—add a bit of water to a maxi-pad and place it in your freezer. Just be sure to place a tissue or washcloth over the pad when you use it.

Rest: Make a little nest or two, probably on your bed and on the living room couch. You'll want a few good pillows, a glass of water and some snacks, maybe your phone and a book and—yes, definitely your baby, too.

And then stay there. With your legs together.

For at least one week, and even better two.

Okay, you're allowed up to pee (see above re: squirt bottle) and bathe and eat and also to breathe some outside air. But really and truly try to think of the first two weeks postpartum as two weeks of rest.

So many people try to do it all right away. They're at the supermarket and they're at the park and they're lugging around the pop-out car seat and they're saying, I'm fine, I'm great, look at how normal I am.

They may be holding it all together, but their lives are not normal. Have reverence for all your body has done and is still doing. Stay home. Ask for help. Rest. You cannot heal at four or six or twelve weeks the way you can heal now, when the tissue is raw and ready to knit together. If you keep worrying a wound, it scars.

There will be time to be that woman: at the park, in the sun, with your baby.

This is your time to rest and heal, feed and sleep.

Let your body heal. You will heal.

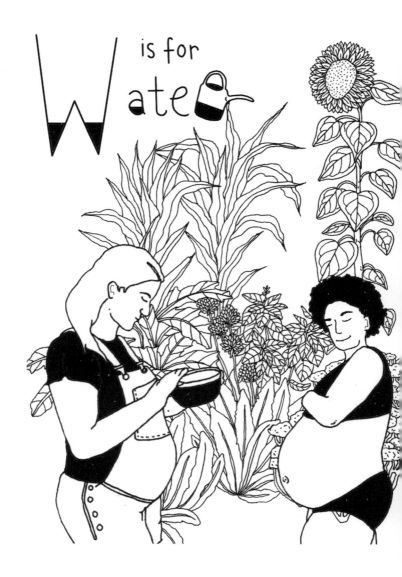

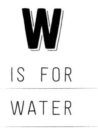

IS FOR

WATER

Annika is on her hands and knees, pushing. Her husband stands on one side of her, holds her hair so it doesn't slip into her face—he can't find the hairband she'd packed, and she's too close now to care. Her sister is on her other side, crying already. Annika's water hasn't yet broken, and as she pushes it looks like a snow globe coming into view: the round membrane filled with water, the flecks of vernix floating within. And then the time for pushing gives way to panting, and slowly, slowly Annika's body opens, her baby's head is born, the shoulders rotate and deliver, and her baby slips from inside to outside and enters our world.

Annika gazes down at her baby, considering this creature still perfectly enclosed in the amniotic sac: elbows and knees bent to her belly, hands clenched beside her head. For one moment Annika looks, and then, for the first time—and yet as if she has done it one hundred times—she reaches for her baby, brings her to her chest. As Annika sits back on her heels we gently wipe the membranes from the baby's face, and as Annika bends to kiss her baby's head the newborn mouth opens, the fists un-furl, and she cries out: a perfect, pinkening newborn cry.

And now even I have to blink away the tears.

For all the births I've been at, I've only seen two ba-bies born in the caul. Usually the amniotic sac ruptures at some point in the labor process, the "water breaking" prior to the baby's arrival. Sometimes it breaks before la-bor begins (this is Hollywood's favorite birth trope, inev-itably followed by a shot of our heroine screaming while being wheelchair-rushed down a hospital corridor), and sometimes we might recommend artificially rupturing the membranes—meaning, the care provider breaks the wa-ter. Doing so can increase the strength of contractions, if augmentation is needed; as with so many other aspects of labor and delivery, just because we can "do" something doesn't mean we should, and unless there's a compelling reason to artificially rupture the membranes, we shouldn't.

I remember floating in the ocean while pregnant with my first baby; it felt comforting and connecting to imag-ine her floating inside me at the same time. Swimming is healthy throughout pregnancy—is there a safer, lower-impact form of exercise?—and though the studies aren't all that convincing, old wives' tales hold that diving into handstands might just turn a stubborn breech.

Water immersion is a great labor trick as well; studies show that women who labor in water experience less dis-comfort. I am forever leading clients to the shower or tub, where they can labor in a dark, calm environment for . . . well, for as long as the hot water lasts. Some clients are interested in water birth, and some hospitals even offer this option. There's lots of controversy about whether birth in water is as safe as birth on land—if you're interested, ask your care provider about his experience with water birth.

(One last plug for all things water: make it your constant drink during pregnancy. Juice is packed with sugar that quickly hits your bloodstream—and then passes through the placenta to your baby. Soda is, of course, even worse. Growing a baby is thirsty work, and water is the best drink for it.)

Back to Annika, and her marvelously intact membranes. After the birth, I told her how rare caul deliveries are and shared that in many cultures being born in the caul is a sign of good luck. Annika herself was an English professor, so of course I felt the need to provide a literary reference: Charles Dickens's David Copperfield. "I was born with a caul," Copperfield tells us in the opening pages of his apparent autobiography, "which was advertised for sale, in the newspapers, at the low price of fifteen guineas."

Annika opted not to sell her daughter's caul, instead burying it alongside the placenta in her tiny backyard. Her sister planted a small fig tree above the spot, and to the best of my knowledge it is there today, growing taller and stronger each year, well cared for—and well watered.

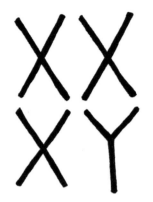

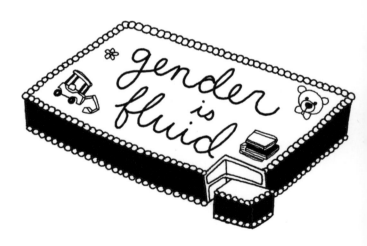

XX/XY

"Do you know what you're having?" everyone—and by that I mean really everyone—asks.

Vera knows she's having a girl: she asked us to put the information in an envelope for her, as our local ultrasound facility won't tell clients directly. She gave the envelope to her mother, who baked a cake. When she and her husband cut into it, they both started crying when they saw the bright pink inside.

Marta and Julia didn't want to know. At the birth, Julia helps me catch their baby and, weeping, lifts her baby into Marta's waiting arms. A nurse covers the baby with a warm blanket, rubs the baby's back. The baby responds with lusty cries—is any sound so wonderful as the cry of a newborn baby?—and Marta and Julia hold each other, overcome. It isn't until the baby is a few minutes old that they pull back the blanket, discover with delight: it's a boy.

Before our children are born we have the chance to know: boy or girl. People generally talk about finding out the gender of their babies, but technically a baby's anatomy refers to the baby's sex: gender is socially constructed, learned behavior, and speaks to what a child identifies as rather than what parts a child was born with.

In my first pregnancy, we opted to learn the sex of our baby from ultrasound; in my subsequent two, we decided to wait. Each time I'd thought I was having a boy; after the birth of my second daughter, I realized my intuition was somewhat lacking. Our third child was born during a blue-sky morning in early June; his sisters, aged six and eight, announced his sex for us. I surprised myself by feeling completely unsurprised—so here he was, at last.

Yet in the days after my son's birth I realized how much of my identity as a mother had been as a mother of girls. When I met my daughter's classmates, it was the girls whose names I remembered—the boys had always looked the same to me, a blur of shaggy hair and blue sweatpants.

Now one of those blurry-boys would be my own.

Some gender differences do assert themselves early. As other mothers had warned me he would, my son turned everything into a gun: sticks, water bottles, and, perhaps strangest of all, a plastic sword. He loved trucks and made me read him the same mind-numbingly boring board book about diggers over and over again. Ever original, he announced he'd be a fireman when he grew up.

"Fire fighter," I corrected him.

"Fireman," he insisted and ran off to shoot some ferns with his water bottle.

I got a kick out of the boy stuff—it was new for me, and it was curious to note how naturally he gravitated toward stereotypically "male" gendered toys and traits in a way the girls had not. But it also got me thinking: Was I noticing the ways in which he was different from his sisters and discounting all the ways in which he was similar?

Like his older sisters, he'll bring me a pile of books and snuggle close as we read each one. Like his older sisters, he likes forest walks and beach hunts and hours and hours of imaginative play. He gravitates toward Lego whereas the girls populated their worlds with stuffed animals, and perhaps there's a bit more bad-guy-vanquished-by-superhero-type action, but his imaginative world, like theirs, tests the boundaries of chaos against the reemergence of order.

So far, my son seems to identify as a boy—and his sisters continue to identify as girls. I recognize that this could change, and that if it did, it would shift my identity, too. And yet: I also know that though the moment when we discovered the sex of each child stays with us, that moment was about my discovery—not my children's.

One of the pleasures of parenting is simply watching as your child's personality unfolds, as they become who they were meant to be. Whether you're told your baby's sex during a second-trimester ultrasound or wait to discover it on the big birth day, it's still worth remembering: there's so much more than that to learn about your baby. Just keep an open mind. Your children will show you, in time, who they are.

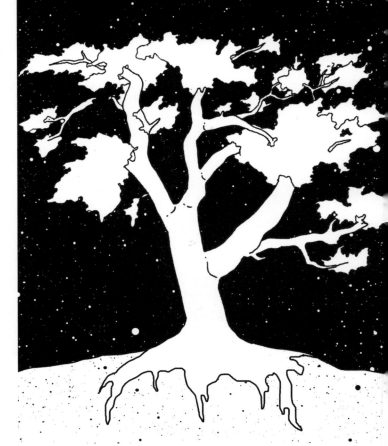

Z

IS FOR

ZEST

I had been present for hundreds of births before I witnessed my first death.

My father called me on the day that he was told that further cancer treatment was no longer recommended, and that likely he had only a few months to live.

"Listen," he said, "what matters: I love you, and I love the way that you're raising your children."

It sounded so simple.

But in the end, it's everything, isn't it?

In the early hours of a November morning, my father died in the same Brooklyn home where I'd been raised. From the moment of his diagnosis, I had worried that, living so far away, I wouldn't be there for the end. I continue to be grateful that I was; even in dying, he taught me so much.

My father had a zest for life. When people say things like that, they sometimes mean that the person engaged in extraordinary activities: they hiked Mount Everest, maybe, or kayaked off Patagonia. I don't mean anything like that at all. My father, a physician, loved his work. He loved his city. He loved finding a good parking spot, reading the Sunday *New York Times*, watching sports, and debating politics. He loved food and drink and good company. For him, eating—by which I mean devouring, with relish, a good meal—was a metaphor for living. He had, as they say, an appetite for life.

This world is bookended by two portals: birth and death. Watching my father die, I felt so grateful to the midwives, nurses, and doctors who had taught me how to sit with laboring women, how to hold space. Death, after all, is a labor, too, and one that, like birth, takes place on its own, unknowable time line. Watching my father die, I felt grateful for the privilege of a life's work immersed in birth, which time and again allows me to witness moments of strength, grace, beauty, and joy:

At a clinic visit, a client lies back, eyes on the ceiling as I move the fetal Doppler over her abdomen, try to hear the fetal heart rate for the first time. I see her close her eyes, bite her lip—she and I have been here before and have been met with silence. This time: the unmistakable horse gallop of the fetal heart. She starts crying and ends laughing, dabbing the tissue to the corner of her eyes, giddy with happiness and relief.

In the midst of a long labor induction, a young woman sits cross-legged on a hospital bed. She breathes through the contractions, her neck flushed, her hand on her belly. Her sister sits behind her, runs a brush through her hair, plaits it into a long braid that hangs heavy down her back.

During a cesarean section, a husband locks eyes with his wife. They hold each other's gaze as the surgery begins, as the workaday rhythm of the operating room unfolds around them, as their baby is lifted from her body.

Visiting a new parent at home at one week postpartum, I place the baby on our portable scale. The parent leans over me to read the numbers, anxious—feeds have been a struggle, and we've been watching the baby's weight closely. Seeing that their baby has gained four ounces in two days, exceeding our goal, my client raises a triumphant fist in the air, pumps it once, twice, three times. It's a victory of a few ounces, and it's everything. Together, they've made it.

Pregnancy, birth, parenting: none of it is easy.
Embrace it all, anyway.
Grow with it.
In the end, it's what matters.

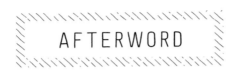

AFTERWORD

Layla smiled at me, shook her head. "You don't know my story," she said to me.

I looked at her, surprised. Just a few weeks into my midwifery studies, my professor had suggested I get to know clients by asking them general, open-ended questions. "How do you feel about your pregnancy?" I'd asked Layla.

Layla had started to answer, and then paused. And that's when she told me: "You don't know my story."

And I didn't.

So she shared it with me.

When we met, Layla was six months pregnant with her second child. Her first child had been born just a few months after she'd arrived in Canada. "My husband and I . . . ," she told me, searching for the right words. "It's not like what you think about arranged marriage. We do love each other. But we didn't know each other that well." She'd had a long labor, and a difficult delivery. Afterward, she felt isolated and alone in her suburban apartment; her husband was at work all day, her family and friends tens of thousands of miles away.

She went to a doctor and had an IUD placed. "I was so depressed," she told me. "I didn't want another baby ever."

Time passed. Her daughter began to crawl, and then walk. She took her to the nearby playground, and there she met other women, immigrants like her.

One day one of them told her a story: another friend had just found out she was pregnant. "And she had an IUD!" the woman confided, eyes wide.

Layla made another appointment with her doctor. Her doctor examined her and reassured her: the IUD was well placed, she was protected.

That very month, Layla missed her period.

"At first I was upset," Layla admitted. "But now I'm okay. I have friends, my daughter has friends. It won't be like before." She looked at me, smiled again. "So, that's my story."

I have thought back to that encounter many, many times over the years.

Up until that conversation, I'd thought that in leaving my previous work as a writer and editor to become a midwife I'd undergone a massive career change. When Layla told me her story—when she framed it for me as "her story"—I understood that while the details of my work had drastically changed, something essential remained the same.

Women's stories would remain the focus of my work.

People speak of midwifery as a calling. There's a part of me that always finds that a bit heavy-handed, and in truth I look forward to a future where a career in midwifery will be viewed just like any career in medicine: incredibly challenging, constantly rewarding, always respected.

Instead, the revelation that I'm a midwife still sometimes leads to eyebrow-raised didn't-we-burn-you-at-the-stake queries.

(True story: I once told a cabdriver I was studying midwifery.

"Midwifery?" he asked, "What is that?"

I explained that we cared for pregnant women and babies.

The driver thought for a bit, then ventured that those women must get really fat.

I was taken aback. "Excuse me?"

"Well," he explained, "pregnant women get fat anyway. But if you're doing all their cooking and cleaning while they lay around—"

"No, no," I said, interrupting. "We provide clinical care." I paused, then stated the obvious. "Like a doctor," I told him.

"Oh," he said, laughing. "I guess it was the word 'wife' that confused me."

Yikes.)

In my own life, midwifery did indeed feel a bit like a calling. Which is a good thing, given the many sleepless nights and high-stress moments—had I chosen it for purely practical reasons, I would never have gotten through the training. I didn't choose midwifery because I thought it'd offer a reasonable work-life balance or even because I thought it spoke to my strengths. I chose midwifery because it merged, for me, my interests in medicine and feminism, and because, on a very basic level, I wanted work that had meaning, work that, as simple as it sounds, would make the world a better place.

Midwifery does.

Here's how it called me.

First knock: I'm a young child, in a nightgown. I stand in the doorway of the living room in our Brooklyn home, watch the big-bellied pregnant women take deep breaths in, release deep breaths out. My mother, a nurse and a Lamaze instructor, stands at the front of the room. "Hoo hoo hoo," she says, her mouth a perfect O as she demonstrates breathing for second stage, "ha ha ha." The light in the room is dim; it is past my bedtime. I watch the women as they watch my mother. Something serious is happening, something sacred.

Second knock: I'm an undergraduate living in Manhattan, studying European history. I come across a short profile in our campus newspaper of an alumna studying midwifery. I read it several times. You can study midwifery? It still exists? I wish, suddenly, that I'd pursued a premed track so I could apply to the master's in midwifery program. But I'm a senior—it's too late. I place the paper in a campus recycling bin and hurry to class.

Third knock: My boyfriend and I move to Philadelphia for his graduate studies. His university offers a master's in nurse midwifery, and I meet some of the women in the program. I pepper them with questions; at a party one of them hosts, I spend most of the evening poring over the midwifery texts on her bookshelf, wanting to read each one. "In another life I would have been a midwife," I tell someone.

Fourth and final knock: I marry my boyfriend; together we go and visit his brother in Toronto. His brother's wife is pregnant, and she has a midwife. She tells me that midwifery is free in Ontario, and that with a midwife she can choose to have her baby at home or in the hospital. I return to Philadelphia before their baby arrives, but my husband stays on. Over the phone, he describes a postpartum home visit from the midwife, how she examined our newborn niece, Maia, as she lay on a sun patch on her parents' bed.

"It was so gentle," he tells me.

I remember myself saying, "In another life I'd have been a midwife."

What about this life? I ask myself.

In Canada, midwifery is a four-year undergraduate degree. I decide to apply, reassuring myself that they won't accept me.

Six years and two babies of my own later, I become a Registered Midwife.

Things I love about Canadian midwifery:

Getting to know clients over the course of their pregnancy. Watching a woman's belly grow, listening as her questions change as her pregnancy progresses. Receiving the page that she is in labor, a familiar voice on the phone—we know each other.

Calling my hospital to alert them to a home birth in progress, or completed, or even that I'm transferring my client to the hospital from home. After all: a birth that begins at home and ends in the hospital isn't a "failed" home birth—it's evidence of a system working well, where women are triaged appropriately.

Visiting families at home in the early days after a birth. Providing breastfeeding support in a woman's own space; discussing safe sleep in the context of her own bedroom.

Evaluating, reassuring. Watching as women come into motherhood, witnessing their confidence grow.

And a final moment, present only by its absence: hugging families good-bye at their final visit and watching them leave, knowing no financial bill follows them out; all my services, from the first intake to the final visit, are covered by our province's medical care plan.

As care providers, we play a powerful role in women's stories. We are actors, interpreters, witnesses. Our role is important; those roles are important.

But it is not our story to title. It is not our story to tell.

"You don't know my story," Layla had said to me.

And then—it amazes me still, the incredible privilege of my work—she shared it with me.

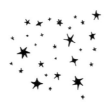

ACKNOWLEDGMENTS

Thank you to my generous readers: Ellen Friedrichs, Joss Hurtig-Mitchell, Dr. Sarah Krotz, Juliet Latham, Luba Lyons, and Paula Schikkerling.

Thank you to the dedicated staff at William Morrow, including Lynn Grady, Cassie Jones, Susan Kosko, Bonni Leon-Berman, Jessica Lyons, Andrea Molitor, Mumtaz Mustafa, Liate Stehlik, and Molly Waxman.

Special thanks to Iris Gottleib, illustrator extraordinaire, for such smart and gorgeous imagery. Heaps of praise to my absolute gem of an editor, Emma Brodie, for thoughtful questions and constant encouragement.

I still can't get over my crazy good luck in successfully wooing Joy Tutela to be my agent. Thank you, Joy, for believing in this project and working your tail off to see it come to fruition. Here's to busy moms-of-three standing up for one another, always. My total gratitude to you and the entire team at David Black Agency Ltd.

Thank you to my incredible midwifery colleagues at my practice, The Midwives Collective in Victoria, British Columbia: Sarah Atkinson, Andrea Dykstra, Jody Medernach, Jill Pearman, and Julia Stolk, along with Julia Young for keeping us all on track. Thank you to all the midwives in the South Island Department of Midwifery, and all the doctors, nurses, and support staff I work alongside at Victoria General Hospital. I am so lucky to have such wise and dedicated colleagues.

Thank you to my husband, Jordan Stanger-Ross, for always cooking dinner. Which is to say: for everything, and not least for being this book's first reader. I am so proud and pleased at the home we have made. When it comes to expressing my thanks to you, and to Eva, Tillie, and Avi, the alphabet becomes inadequate. You all light up my life.

A final thanks to my clients, from whom I have learned so much, for trusting me to be your care provider. Thank you.

YOUR STORY HERE

(fill in name and date)

_____

_____

_____

_____

_____

_____

_____

_____

_____

_____

_____

_____

_____

A IS FOR ADVICE. Copyright © 2019 by Ilana Stanger-Ross. All rights reserved. Printed in China. No part of this book may be used or reproduced in any manner whatsoever without written permission except in the case of brief quotations embodied in critical articles and reviews. For information, address HarperCollins Publishers, 195 Broadway, New York, NY 10007.

HarperCollins books may be purchased for educational, business, or sales promotional use. For information, please email the Special Markets Department at SPsales@harpercollins.com.

FIRST EDITION

WM Morrow Gift is a trademark of HarperCollins

DESIGNED BY BONNI LEON-BERMAN

Library of Congress Cataloging-in-Publication Data has been applied for.

ISBN 978-0-06-283878-0

19 20 21 22 23 SC 10 9 8 7 6 5 4 3 2 1

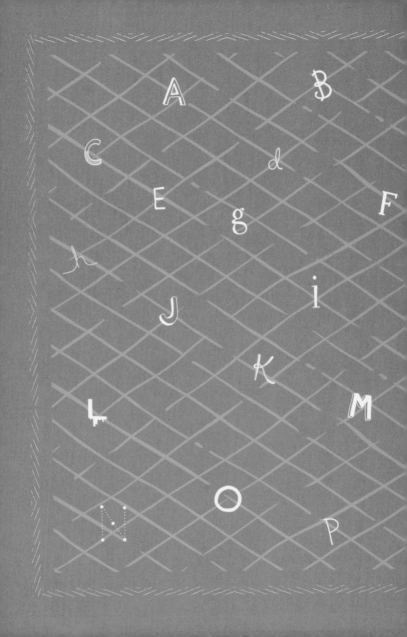